TABLE OF CONTENTS

Your Gift

I wanted to show my appreciation that you support my work so I've put together a free gift for you.

http://bonusfreebook.org/

Just visit the link above to download it now.

I know you will love this gift.

Thank you for attention!

With love,

John Thornton

INTRODUCTION

Despite the fact that most people don't view mornings as a winning time to work-out, it would surprise many how valuable the time is to break a sweat. Many people think about it and maybe even plan for it but never actually get to it. A lot of people have been discovered to take on exercises afternoon rather than do it in the morning. This is so despite the many benefits that may be reaped from morning workouts. According to health and exercise physiologists, every second of the day is precious to workout. Most of the people who love to work-out, however, do it in later hours of the day since they think that they have more time than in the morning hours. This book will be used as a guide for people should wake up to work-out early in the morning. I am sure that people who work-out in the morning are very energetic during their daily activities.

Morning hours contain the least number of distractions and what gets scheduled gets done on most of the occasions. This increases the probability that you will get your workout done during the morning hours. The most prominent advantage is the fact that will get to work-out before you get distracted by other activities. Nothing can get in the way of you and your work-out since you have prioritized it. During the day, so many issues may pop up and distract you but this will be avoided by working out in the morning. One may also be forced to keep on pushing their work-out sessions which will be avoided entirely by doing the work-outs first. The advantages of working out in the morning according to my personal experience lie in the way the body, mind, and soul react. The purpose of this book is to try and bring out the many advantages that lie in working out in the morning and the various ways that the body gains. For people who work out and plans to change the hours of working out in the morning, the book should serve as a perfect and flawless guide to the perfect morning work-outs that will help to start your day fully energized and rejuvenated.

Benefits of Morning Work-out

Working out is limited by the fact that we have to divide the small hours we have during the day among so many things. One will always be forced to opt for work rather than working out in the morning which gives a compelling explanation why most gyms are packed to capacity during after work hours. The purpose of this section is to give a variety of really good reasons explaining why we should wake up a little bit earlier to work-out other than do it during later hours. Right before making excuses as to why you find it difficult to work-out during the morning hours, take your time to go through the many reasons as to why you should sacrifice some morning minutes to hit the gym and carry out that fantastic morning workout session.

1. *Great Hormone Flow to your Advantage*

Powerful hormones that are crucial in the building of those desired muscles are highly raised during the morning hours. Working out in the morning allows us to take full advantage of the naturally circulating hormones when they are at the peak point. Working out during later hours of the day means that the hormones are not raised hence less muscle building will take place. It is thus highly advisable to work-out when the hormones are boosting muscle building for greater benefits.

2. *Creates More Time for Other Duties*

Most of us have so many priorities that we barely have an hour to spare for our bodies which have led to us not working out. This has led to people preferring to spend more time on other priorities like work and family. This is a great reason why one should reduce the hours they spend sleeping especially in the morning to hit the gym. Working out in the morning will then be easier since you don't even have to struggle with the evening hustle and bustle of the rush hour traffic while trying to get that much-needed gym session. The gym is also very crowded in the evening hours and which creates another issue altogether. Everything else will be so much easier to schedule if you can get your workout done in the morning.

3. Systems and Schedules Setup are Easier to Follow

Exercises setup and listed in a training programme are almost impossible to follow in   a packed gym environment. There always seems to be someone who wants to make use of the needed equipment and it always seems as though you are hogging the equipment if you won't share. This does not always play so well at the packed gym. What if you were only two or three people in the same gym that let's say holds about 30-40 people in the evening. Equipment will be at your disposal, and your schedule will be very easy to adhere to. Most people choose to work-out in the evening in almost all scenarios. This will play to your advantage if you decide to work-out in the morning.

4. Increases your Focus Level throughout the Day

Exercising plays the role of arousing your body which increases your focus levels for the next activity. On most occasions, one will probably go to work or go to school after the morning workout session. The advantage, in this case, is that working out will create a high level of alertness and you will be more able to focus on all the day's activities. In any case, most people are too tired after school or after work and sometimes choose to avoid the gym. Wouldn't it be great to work-out and do exceptionally really well during the day? If you are not so energetic in the morning, I would recommend taking pre-workouts that favor your taste, and that will help in focus boosting. The boosters may also boost your strength and energy even after the gym workouts. An example of a pre-workout that I recommend is the Grenade.50 Caliber as shown in the picture below.

5. Fewer Distractions during the Workout

Not so many people want to carry out workout sessions at the break of dawn, and there is a high possibility that you will only do it with a few of your friends who you plan with. If you are serious about working out in the morning, there is a high chance that you will enjoy this. Due to the fewer distractions, you will most likely spend more time working out than socializing and hence reap all the benefits of the morning workout. At the break of dawn, I can bet you that the possibility of other people distracting you during your workouts are minimal hence another superb reason as to you should endeavor to work-out in the morning. In comparison to the evening hours where the gym may be fully packed, working out in the morning may be simply heavenly to people who cherish working out undistracted.

Health Effects of Morning Workouts

The whole reason behind working out is to stay strong and healthy. As years go by, it becomes apparent that the body changes and needs more care. Apart from getting reaped and looking stronger, there are real health benefits and reasons why one should get up early in the morning and workout. It is just not a matter of preference, but a necessity if you want to keep that young feel and look. There are so many benefits that are acquired by simply working out in the morning that it is difficult to exhaust them all. Not only does it improve your daily schedule, but also your health. This next section includes reasons explaining why you should wake up early and work-out.

1. Higher Rate of Burning Fat

Researches indicate when works out on an empty stomach, it helps in burning about 20% more fat than when has had a meal. By the time one wakes up in the morning, most of the food is probably digested. This is another advantage of working out when one wakes up. It will substantially increase the rate at which fat is burned. During the day, one may be tempted to consume a variety of foods, and when it comes to the workouts, the stomach will probably be full. According to the British Journal of Nutrition, it is better to exercise on an empty stomach to burn more fat.

2. Great Way of Protecting Yourself against Diabetes

Working out in the morning before having a meal helps in protecting a person against insulin resistance and glucose intolerance. These are the most significant trademarks of Type 2 diabetes. When one exercise before intake of carbohydrates according to the Journal of Physiology, glucose tolerance and insulin sensitivity are highly improved, and it also helps one not gain weight.

3. Enhanced Metabolism

It has been proved, and it's quite common to hear of EPOC (Excess Post-Exercise Oxygen Consumptions) in the fitness world. This subject its essence simply tries to explain that the body burns more calories after working out no matter what you are doing after even if it's sitting down. This means, exercising in the morning contains a lot of healthy benefits. Even if you eat later on in the day, the higher metabolic rate means that your body will be able to replenish itself at a faster and more effective rate.

4. Improved Mental and Physical Energies

Many of us need a lot of energy to kick off our morning. One of the greatest sources of energy is movement. Working out in the morning has also been shown as one of the many ways of improving focus levels and mental capabilities. Working out in the morning will ensure that you are focused, full of energy and performing at full mental capacity throughout the day. Hitting the iron early in the morning will wake you up better than a cup of coffee. This is because all senses including the body are fully energized once you get your workout going and the impacts will be felt positively throughout the day.

5. Helps you to Sleep Better at Night

I believe that this does not need so much reasoning. It is simple and clear, working out in the morning will help you sleep longer and deeper than working out in the evening. This is attributed to the fact that evening workouts increase body stimulation and temperature which makes sleeping very difficult. On the other hand, working out in the morning creates the desire to sleep as soon as you rest your body on that comfortable bed. The benefits of a good night's rest are well known to all of us.

6. Keeps You Energized all Day Long

This is one of the best facts about working out in the morning. Nothing sucks like a long day at the office feeling all lazy and sickly or even sleepy due to lack of that ounce of energy. In my opinion, it is just not good for you nor is it healthy. Compare it to that guy at the office who is energetic, focused and happy because they worked out in the morning. It is a matter of choice and how you want to feel, but I believe it is better to take that morning workout.

Mistakes in the Training Process

Taking on morning exercises merely is one of the best things that you can do for your health, and the benefits are well known throughout the fitness world. Not only does it reduce risks like heart disease, diabetes, cancer and boost energy levels, it is also very crucial in the management and control of weight. It is, however, no use exercising if you cannot do it right since even the best of intentions may prove fruitless in the long run if the right measure and processes are not undertaken. Below is a list of common mistakes that we tend to make in the morning workouts which may reduce the fruits we reap from this good practice.

- Sacrificing sleep to work-out. You do not need to sacrifice your rest to exercise in the morning. You need to work-out in the correct way over a short period.

- Only working in a single area of the body.

- Not following a suitable program and supporting every piece of advice that you spot thinking that it will work better.

- Overworking the body in the more hoping to achieve better results which have been proven to do more harm than good.

- Not knowing your limits and capabilities which may lead to one over or underestimating their abilities. This may lead to injuries or derail progress.

CHAPTER 1: BASICS

1. Program

- Wake up at a suitable time. Do not wake up so early that you sacrifice your sleep, but early enough to get something done.

- Warm up. Warming up is very important before taking on any type of exercise. Warm up exercises may include any exercises that are not so strenuous but serve the purpose of getting you and your body into the "mood". Just like many activities, morning workouts need some preparation before getting started.

- Strength exercises. This should include any and all exercises that increase your body strength. The purpose of doing them right after warming up is the fact that your body is still energetic and in a position to take on the rigorous strength exercises.

- Endurance exercises. This should be done after the strength exercise just to make ensure that your body is pushed to its ability. You should carry out the endurance exercises to the point that your body is fully worked for the day.

- Cooldown. We can also call this stretching. This should be made up of exercises that are light and relaxing to the body after the tiresome workout. You should make ensure that you have properly cooled down or muscles that have been involved during the workout to avoid any risk of post-workout injuries.

2. Rules

In order to achieve the best results while performing any activity, a variety of rules, regulations and guidelines need to be followed to attain the best possible results. In most cases, the rules work in order to ensure the safety of the person performing the activity and those in their vicinity. In some instances for example for the purpose of the morning workout, the rules will act as a guideline and morale booster towards the activity. The rules will also play their traditional role of ensuring your safety during the workouts as well as throughout the day. As you will see below, in order to achieve maximum results when working out, you need to follow some dos and don'ts.

- Form a habit. Working out this morning and not doing it for the rest of the week is a big NO. Consistency is a must if you want to benefit from the tiresome activity that is working out. It is better to take on a small workout activity each morning than to skip working out due to taking on hard exercises.

- Relax as you work-out all parts of your body. Avoid being tense as you work-out in the morning. Tension leads to waste of energy. Better results will be achieved if you relax the muscles you are not working on and focus on what you are doing to save energy.

- Create a proper routine. Try and work-out all parts of your body by creating a routine that is variable. Never stick to the same exercise over and over on the different days. Try and follow a routine that basically works on all your body. It is easier to do the latter but not exactly beneficial since you need your whole body to reap the benefits of the morning work-outs.

- Create a good diet that will help you grow even as you work-out. Avoid eating as much as you work-out otherwise you will deal with weight issues, Instead find a healthy balanced diet that will be beneficial and contribute to your workouts.

- Choose the right kind of footwear and sportswear and do not wear clothing just because it is trendy. Comfort as you work-out in the morning is of essence. It is very difficult to work-out if you are not comfortable especially in the morning hours and it may lead to you not working out at all.

- Always make sure that you balance your workouts. Do not focus on specific kinds of exercise or muscles and ignore the rest. Balance is essential to fully enjoy the benefits of working out.

3. Nutrition

Good feeding habits are a must to attain that great feel and be healthy at the same time. On most occasions for most people, it is very hard to stomach food early in the morning and some of us barely have the time to even do so. If you do not feel the pangs of hunger at dawn, it is not really necessary to eat anything before your workout. However, if you need to eat something before your workout, you should at least have a clue what to eat before the early morning session. The foods can be taken as recovery snacks or even to energize the body since they are rich in protein and carbs. They are also easy to prepare and do not take too much time. Here is the list.

- ✓ Peanut butter (1/2 tsp.) with a banana
- ✓ Chocolate milk
- ✓ Dried fruits
- ✓ Fruit juice
- ✓ Hardboiled egg and a slice of toast
- ✓ Cereal (a handful)

You can eat the following after the workout or later in the morning.

- ✓ Low fat milk with oatmeal
- ✓ Smoothie (spinach, protein powder, frozen fruit, almond milk or milk).
- ✓ Toast with jam
- ✓ Lentil soup

CHAPTER 2:
WARM UP

As it has been established, waking up early in the morning to work-out is a major issue for many people. This is, in essence, a great reason why we should always try to get our bodies in the mood to work-out. Many are the benefits that are involved with warming up that it would take an entire section to exhaust them. Some of these benefits include injury prevention, mood activation, and to get the blood flowing. This part of your work-out session has positive effects on the body and is also a great safety precaution. The session also prepares the mind and body for the intensive activities that follow. Below are some great warm-up exercises. I believe in really getting the blood pumping hence some of the warm-ups are intense but great for the morning session.

1. The Stretch Warm-Up

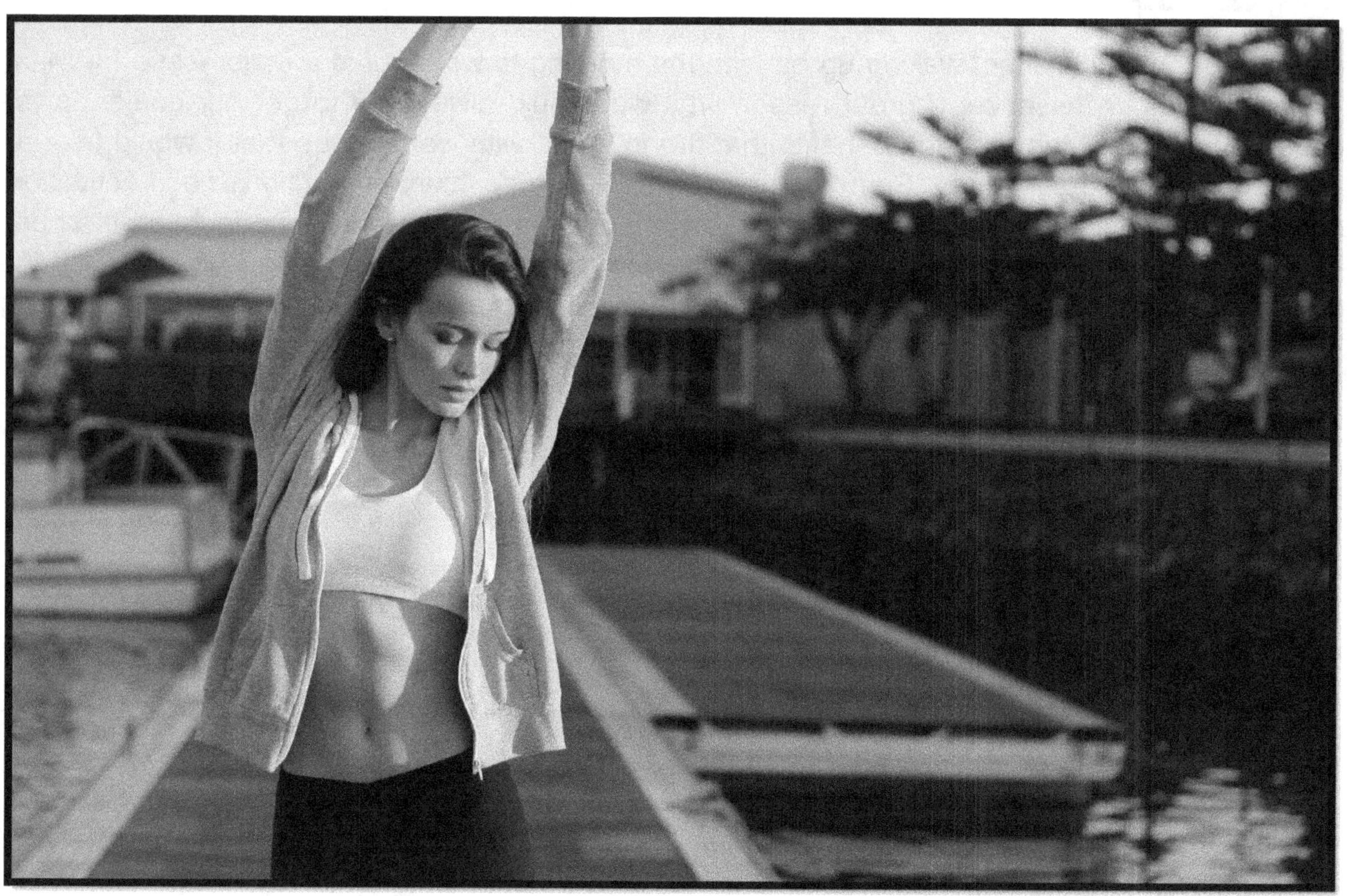

After waking up early in the morning, it is paramount to get the muscles warm right before you get to stretching. Muscles can be greatly strained by morning stretches due to the fact that the night was full of inactivity. To get our blood going and those muscles warm, start by the mere act of walking around the house. Move your hands and legs by shaking them to get that blood flowing and then start your stretching routine after you feel warm enough.

2. Jump rope

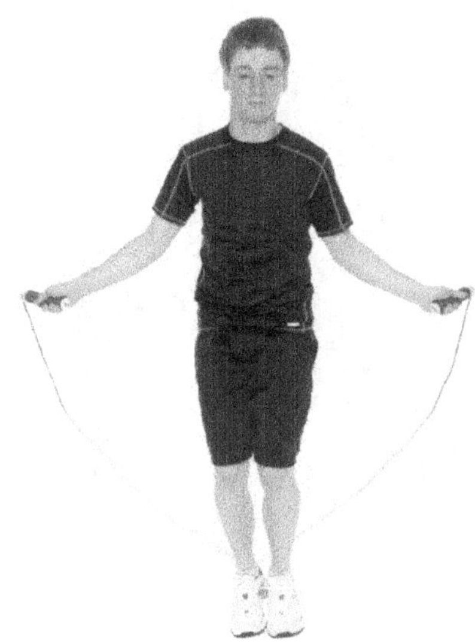

This is a simple exercise that will really get you in the mood. All you need is a skipping rope and you are good to go. Jump the rope for 2-3 minutes and your blood will be as hot as you like it. Do not tire yourself too much since this is only meant for warming up.

3. Jumping Jacks

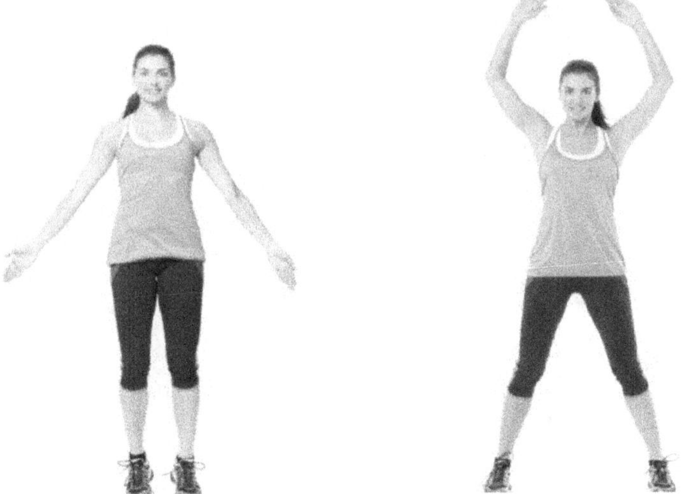

Remember this all-time playtime game with our friends? It is really a good way to warm up.

- Place your hands on your hips

- Stand at attention

- Jump up with your legs widely parted and your hands clapping above your head

- Ensure you land in the initial position

- Repeat 20 times

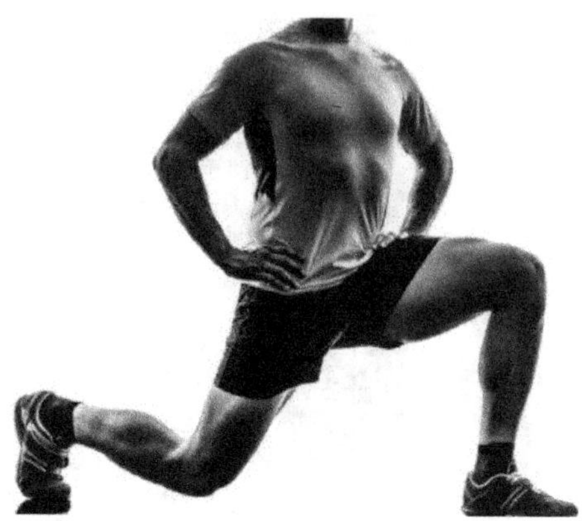

This is another great way to warm up:

- Place your hand on your hips.

- Move one foot forward and let the remaining knee touch the floor as shown in the photo

- Move forward as you perform the lunges

- Make at least 20 while interchanging the legs

5. Squats

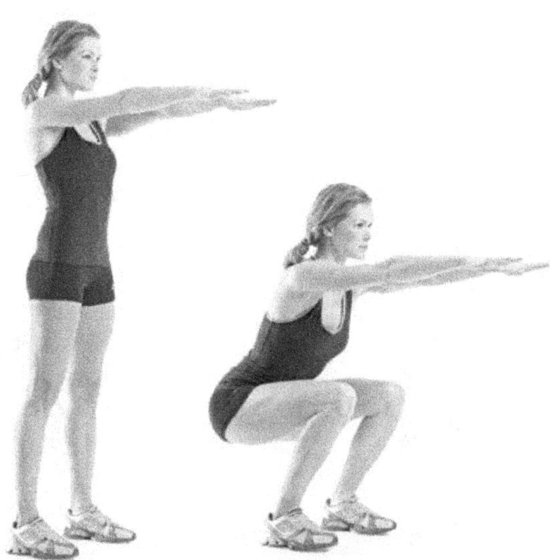

Squats if well done will not only warm you up. They will also strengthen your back and leg muscles. You can choose how to do them but I recommend the following techniques.

- Place your hands in front of your chest at a right angle to your body or place them criss-cross against your chest

- Perform the squats imitating a standing toddler

- You can also spread your legs a little bit

- Do at least 20 of this in the morning to get warmed up.

CHAPTER 3:
STRENGTH EXERCISES

Are you feeling tired of doing the same strength exercises each day? Do you feel like your body is used to the exercises and there is no challenge anymore? Tony Gentlicore, a famous strength coach asserts that the body can adapt to very high amounts of stress when put through it regularly. This is why someone feels like there is no challenge anymore after the same exercises for a long time. In order to realize changes and growth, you need to challenge your muscles every once in a while. This is referred to as the overload principle. By challenging the muscles, I mean adding the number of sets and reps you are used to. In order to challenge the body, you might also decide to take fewer rests and add some weight for the lifts.

Tweaking the exercises is also another very sure way of challenging your body to go further. This keeps the muscles guessing. Luckily, there are ways that you can spice up your daily routine strength exercises like chest press, back squats and bent over rows. Here is how you can spice up your normal exercise to make them more challenging. These exercises can do wonders when done in the morning.

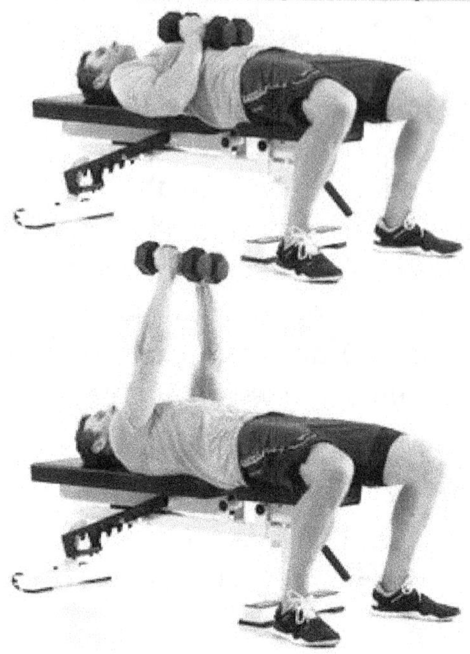

Squeezing two dumbbells together as you do the chest press tremendously increases your time under pressure and tension. This boosts your shoulders and pecks. This is how to perform the squeeze press.

- The best position is by laying on a bench, with the back flat against it, dumbbells held at chest, arms bent and your palms looking away from the face.

- Keep pressing the dumbbells' ends together actively.

- Keep squeezing and pressing the ends together with dumbbells straight over the chest.

- Bring down the weights slowly as you control it and your elbows should dip below the height of the bench slightly.

- Bring the dumbbells up again and keep doing it slowly as you control and feel the weight to realize results.

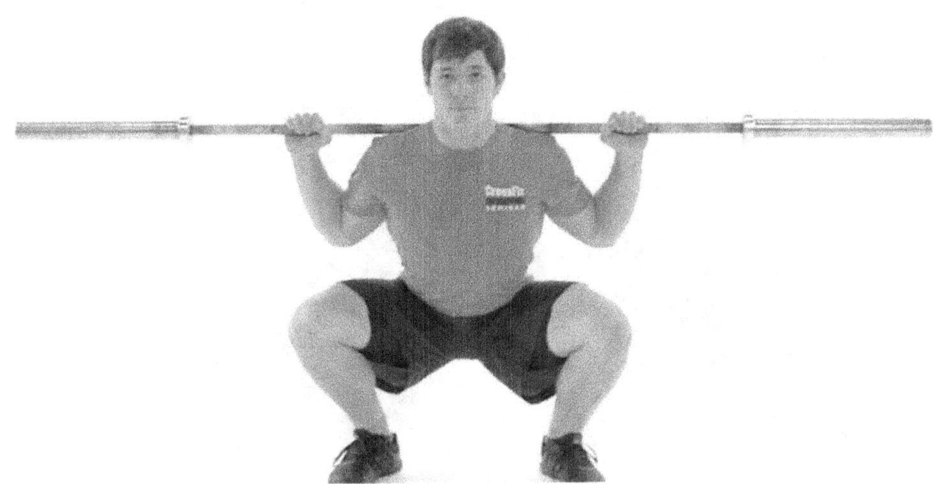

Taking pauses at the bottom of the back squats intensely engages the core and glutes. This is because you keep the back straight and keep up tension at the bottom. This is how to do the back squats with a pause.

- Initiate you squat by bending the knees and lowering downwards with a barbell across your shoulders.

- Keep tension by taking a five seconds pause at the bottom of every squat.

- To push back and stand to engage your heels.

- Throughout the exercise, you should keep your torso straight and knees in line with the toes.

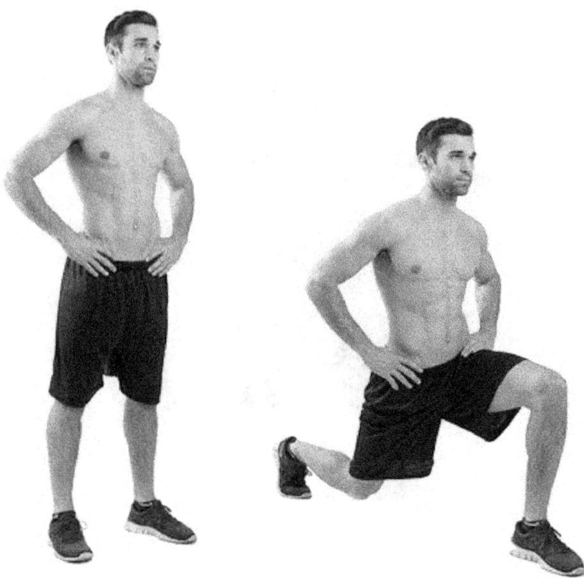

This exercise is good for maintaining balance. It also tests your coordination as you do the movements from a position to the other. This is done while standing on one leg. This is how to perform this strength exercise.

- Stand with legs apart (shoulders width). Take a step forward with one foot and go down from your hips with control towards the ground.

- Go back to standing position by engaging the heel of your front foot.

- In the standing position take one big step behind with the front legs.

- Do the lowering manoeuver again.

- Keep repeating as you switch sides.

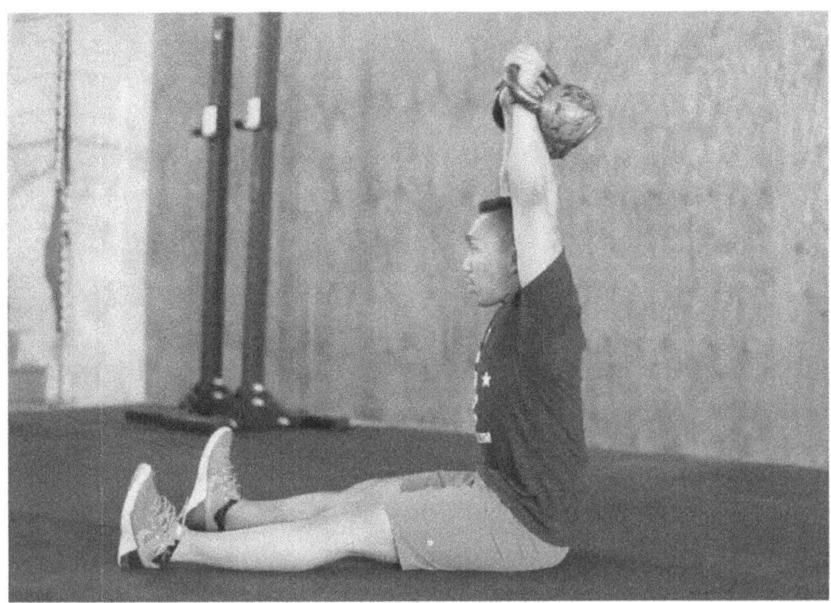

Taking this exercise on the floor engages the muscles more than when seated. Doing it on the floor engages the hips more than when seated. This is how to perform the z presses.

- Get two dumbbells and et a barbell low to a point you can press overhead when seated on the floor.

- Extend legs in a v shape as you're seated. While seated tall press the dumbbells overhead with heels and legs pressed against the ground.

- With control lower the weight again until shoulder length repeatedly.

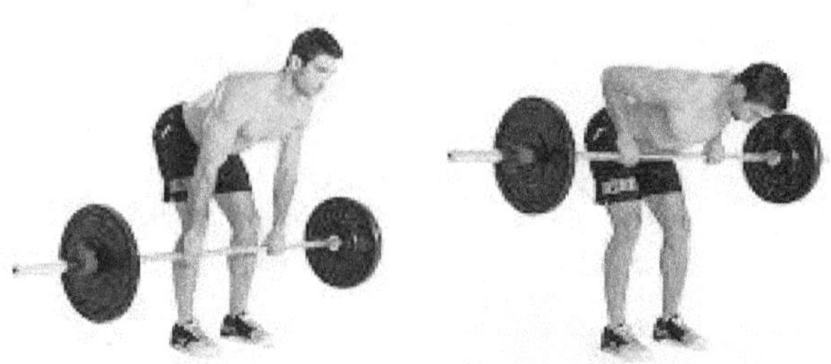

Grip position can either make an exercise harder or easier. By getting more comfortable positions you can be able to work more and achieve more. This is how to perform this exercise:

- With an overhand grip, keep your chest up and chin down while pulling the barbell towards the ribcage, elbows pulled back towards the hips. Stop at the midline. At the top of the movement squeeze the shoulder blades.

- Lower barbell control. Without breaking down perform as many reps as possible. When you start to feel tension on muscles switch to an underhand grip.

6. Instead of crunches try the reverse crunches

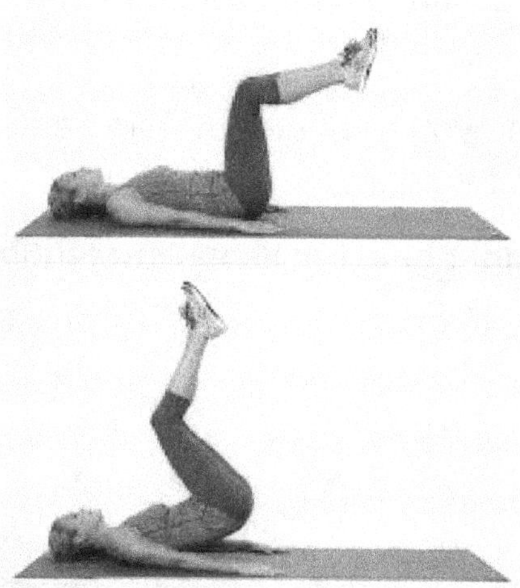

Reverse crunches build your lower abs. reverse crunches also reduce taxing on spine. This is how to perform the reverse crunches.

- Lie on your back and bend knees at ninety degrees. Fingertips rest at the back of the head. Keep chest open and elbows wide.

- Bring knees towards the chest and lift butt from the floor.

- Lower hips slowly with control back to start position.

CHAPTER 4: ENDURANCE EXERCISE

Endurance exercises help the body to withstand vigorous movement for a long time. Endurance allows the body to execute many actions at a single time for a longer period of time. The exercise discussed below will greatly assist in increasing your endurance.

1. Squat jumps

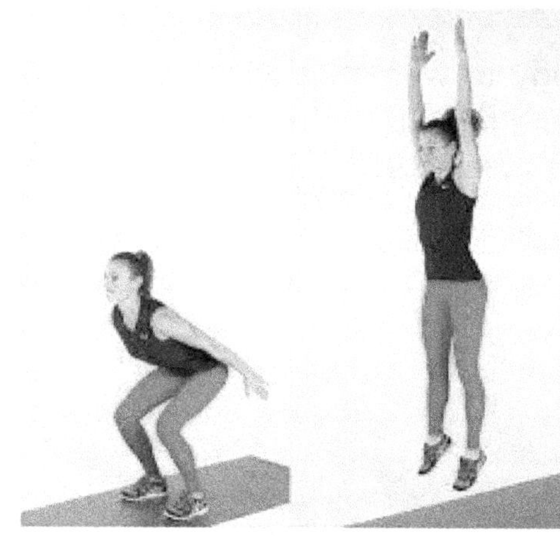

They challenge thighs, hips and glutes. How to do it:

- Stay at a squat position.

- Ensure you are upright.

- Push yourself to explode upwards repeatedly.

2. Box jumps

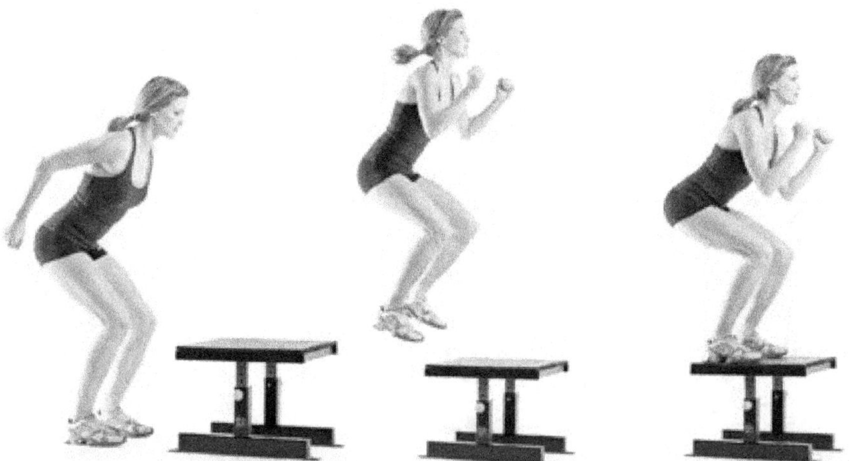

This exercise fires up the quads, glutes and hamstrings. How to do it:

- Stand facing box.

- Bend knees into semi squat position.

- Jump onto the box softly.

- Step back to the floor and continue that movement.

3. Bounding

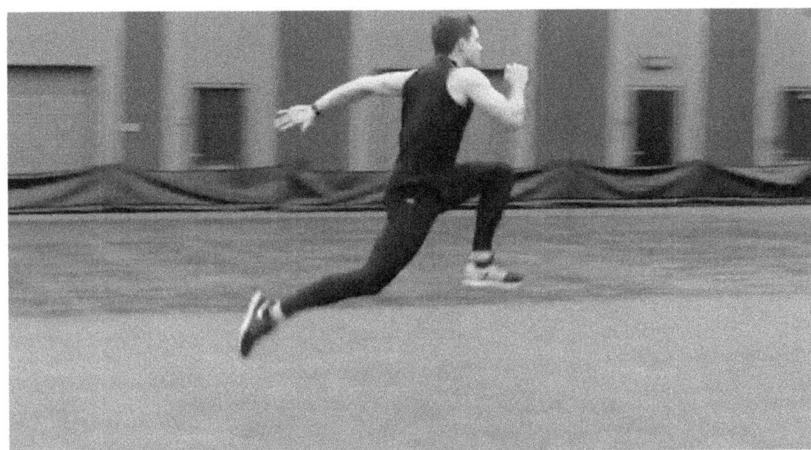

This exercise builds coordination, power and speed. How to do it:

- Start drill by jogging.

- Explode with one foot and bring forward the leg while at the same time pushing the opposite hand forward.т

- Make the running movement exaggerated repeatedly to engage muscles.

4. Power pushups

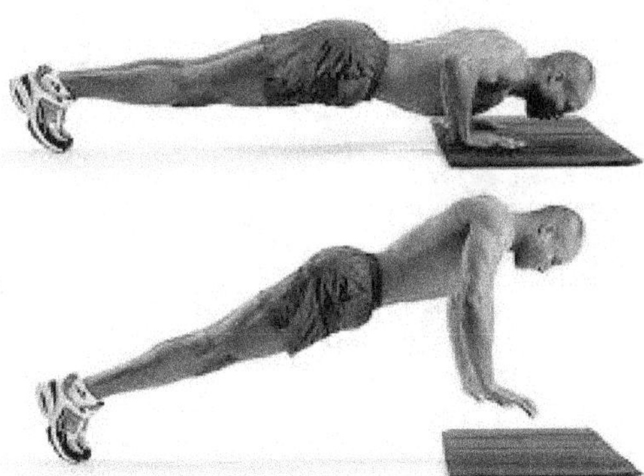

This is basically a pumped up traditional push up. It engages the triceps, chest and shoulders. How to do it:

- Stay in push up position.

- Do the traditional push up but with more force until your hands leave the surface of the ground.

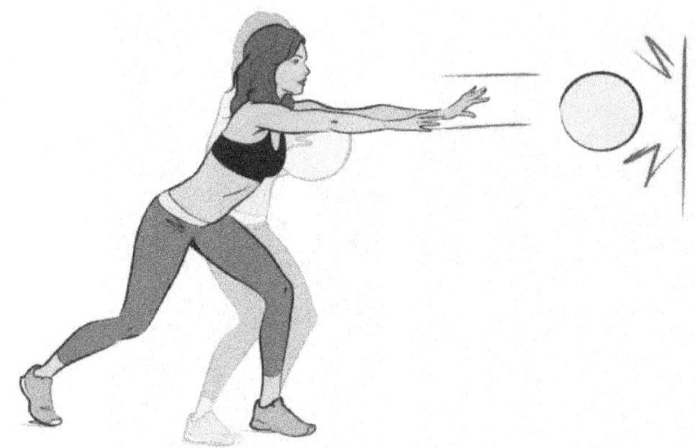

This exercise builds the chest and triceps. How to do it:

- Face a wall with a medicine ball and throw it towards the wall with both hands.

- When it bounces back to throw it again repeatedly.

6. Overhead passes

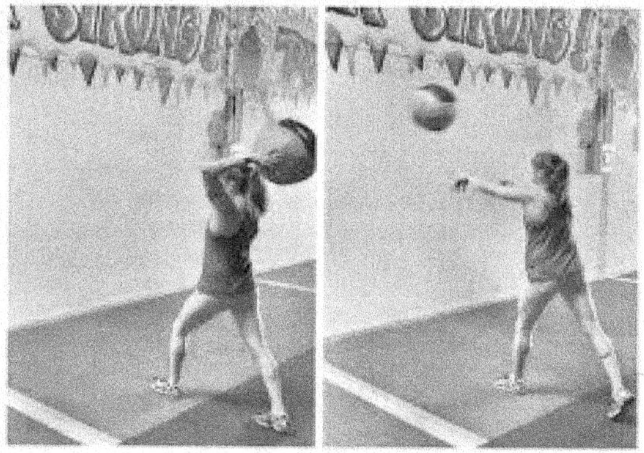

This exercise focuses on the biceps, chest and beck. How to perform the exercise:

- Hold a medicine ball over the head with both hands.

- Throw it far away as possible.

- Keep throwing repeatedly to engage your shoulders and arms.

CHAPTER 5: COOLDOWN

Before every work out you need to do a warm-up and after every work out you need to do a cooldown. Warm ups loosen the body and stretch relax the muscles after a workout. The cooldown strategy described below lasts around 5 minutes but is conclusive. It is convenient for everyone even those people with limited time. The stretches at the cooldown are very essential is bringing down the heart rate after vigorous exercise. This is the work out's structure for the cooldown.

- Do some light cardio to bring the heart rate down and then go into stretches for the other muscles

- Take 15 seconds on every exercise or stretch

- Do the cooldown for around 5 minutes

- The stretches and exercises should range from torso twists, shoulder stretch, glute stretch, toe touch, shoulder rolls and boxer shuffle. This should all be done for around 15 seconds each a period of total 5 minutes

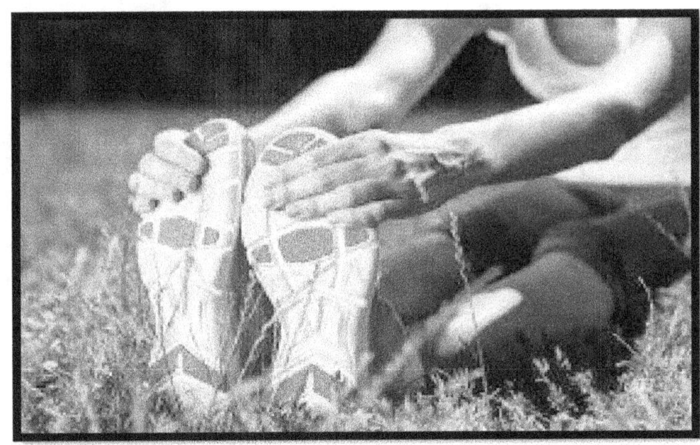

CHAPTER 6:
CONCLUSION

As discussed in the previous chapters, working out in the morning is a great benefit. Not only does it help to improve your health, it also aids the body and mind to cope with the hard activities that make up our hard day to day lives. Done in the right way, morning workouts will not only leave you energized and ready to handle whatever is thrown your way, but they will also leave you looking and feeling great. Like any other form of workout, it is important to make plans and draw up flexible schedules that are easy to follow or it will be even more difficult to get the exercises done. As seen in the first chapters, it is even easier to work out in the morning than in the traditional evening hours. I hope my book will be as a good guide and provide great results in your workouts. Since the book also tries to give nutritional advice, I hope the recommended foods can also work wonders. Don't be a slouch, get up and get moving. Working out is not easy, but looking and feeling fit isn't either. I am however certain that following the chapters closely won`t only give you a great read but will also give great ideas on how to work out.

Your Gift

I wanted to show my appreciation that you support my work so I've put together a free gift for you.

http://bonusfreebook.org/

Just visit the link above to download it now.

I know you will love this gift.

Thank you for attention!

With love,

John Thornton

Legal & Disclaimer